Raja Yoga Explained: Yoga for Beginners Guide

New Step by Step Guide on Raja Yoga

By: Sanjay Tewani

9781631871665

I0413983

PUBLISHER'S NOTES

Disclaimer – Speedy Publishing, LLC

This publication is intended to provide helpful and informative material. It is not intended to diagnose, treat, cure, or prevent any health problem or condition, nor is intended to replace the advice of a physician. No action should be taken solely on the contents of this book. Always consult your physician or qualified healthcare professional on any matters regarding your health and before adopting any suggestions in this book or drawing inferences from it.

The author and publisher specifically disclaim all responsibility for any liability, loss or risk, personal or otherwise, which is incurred as a consequence, directly or indirectly, from the use or application of any contents of this book.

Any and all product names referenced within this book are the trademarks of their respective owners. None of these owners have sponsored, authorized, endorsed, or approved this book.

Always read all information provided by the manufacturers' product labels before using their products. The author and publisher are not responsible for claims made by manufacturers.

This book was originally printed before 2014. This is an adapted reprint by Speedy Publishing LLC with newly updated content designed to help readers with much more accurate and timely information and data.

Speedy Publishing, LLC©2014

40 E. Main St. #1156

Newark, Delaware

19711

Contact Us: 1-888-248-4521

Website: http://www.speedypublishing.com

REPRINTED Paperback Edition: ISBN: 9781631871665

Manufactured in the United States of America

DEDICATION

This book is dedicated to all those who seek the truth about their existence. Inner peace can be achieved, but a higher level of awareness has to be reached. That is just a bit of what Raja yoga can teach you.

TABLE OF CONTENTS

INTRODUCTION - THE CONCEPT OF I

In India, the Candidates for Initiation into the science of "Raja Yoga," when they apply to the Yogi Masters for instruction, are given a series of lessons designed to enlighten them regarding the nature of the Real Self, and to instruct them in the secret knowledge whereby they may develop the consciousness and realization of the real "I" within them. They are shown how they may cast aside the erroneous or imperfect knowledge regarding their real identity.

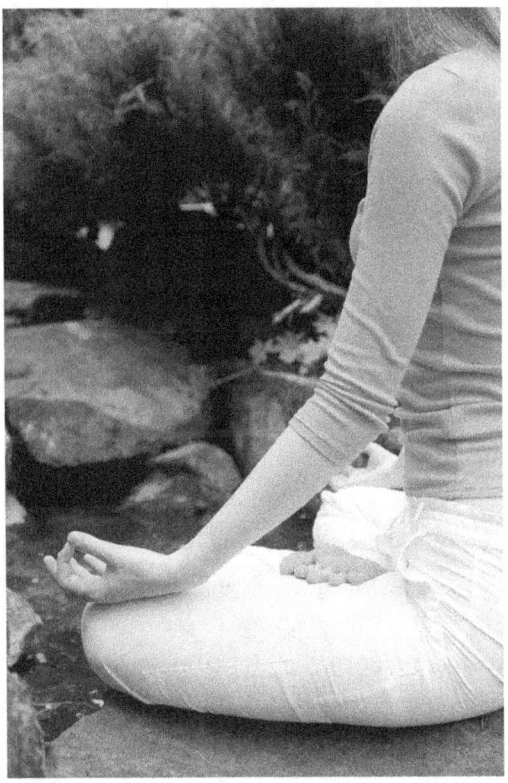

Until the Candidate masters this instruction, or at least until the truth becomes fixed in his consciousness, further instruction is denied him, for it is held that until he has awakened to a conscious realization of his Actual Identity, he is not able to understand the source of his power, and, moreover, is not able to _feel_ within him the power of the Will, which power underlies the entire teachings of "Raja Yoga."

The Yogi Masters are not satisfied if the Candidate forms merely a clear intellectual conception of this Actual Identity, but they insist that he must _feel_ the truth of the same--must become _aware_ of the Real Self--must enter into a consciousness in which the realization becomes a part of his everyday self--in which the realizing consciousness becomes the prevailing idea in his mind, around which his entire thoughts and actions revolve.

To some Candidates, this realization comes like a lightning flash the moment the attention is directed toward it, while in other cases the Candidates find it necessary to follow a rigorous course of training before they acquire the realization in consciousness.

The Yogi Masters teach that there are two degrees of this awakening consciousness of the Real Self. The first, which they call "the Consciousness of the 'I'," is the full consciousness of _real_ existence that comes to the Candidate, and which causes him to _know_ that he is a real entity having a life not depending upon the body--life that will go on in spite of the destruction of the body--_real_ life, in fact. The second degree, which they call "the Consciousness of the 'I AM'," is the consciousness of one's identity with the Universal Life, and his relationship to, and "in-touchness" with all life, expressed and unexpressed. These two degrees of consciousness come in time to all who seek "The Path." To some it comes suddenly; to others, it dawns gradually; to many it comes assisted by the exercises and practical work of "Raja Yoga."

The first lesson of the Yogi Masters to the Candidates, leading up to the first degree, above mentioned, is as follows: That the Supreme Intelligence of the Universe--the Absolute--has manifested the being that we call Man--the highest manifestation on this planet. The Absolute has manifested an infinitude of forms of life in the Universe, including distant worlds, suns, planets, etc., many of these forms being unknown to us on this planet, and being impossible of conception by the mind of the ordinary man. But these lessons have nothing to do with that part of the philosophy which deals with these myriad forms of life, for our time will be taken up with the unfoldment in the mind of man of his true nature and power. Before man attempts to solve the secrets of the Universe without, he should master the Universe within--the Kingdom of the Self. When he has accomplished this, then he may, and should, go forth to gain the outer knowledge as a Master demanding its secrets, rather than as a slave begging for the crumbs from the table of knowledge. The first knowledge for the Candidate is the knowledge of the Self.

Man, the highest manifestation of the Absolute, as far as this planet is concerned, is a wonderfully organized being--although the average man understands but little of his real nature. He comprises within his physical, mental and spiritual make-up both the highest and the lowest, as we have shown in our previous lessons (the "Fourteen Lessons" and the "Advanced Course"). In his bones he manifests almost in the form of mineral life, in fact, in his bones, body and blood mineral substances actually exist. The physical life of the body resembles the life of the plant.

Many of the physical desires and emotions are akin to those of the lower animals, and in the undeveloped man these desires and emotions predominate and overpower the higher nature, which latter is scarcely in evidence. Then, Man has a set of mental characteristics that are his own, and which are not possessed by the lower animals (See "Fourteen Lessons"). And in addition to the mental faculties common to all men, or rather, that are in evidence in a greater or lesser degree among all men, there are still higher faculties latent within Man, which when manifested and expressed render Man more than ordinary Man. The unfoldment of these latent faculties is possible to all who have reached the proper stage of development and the desire and hunger of the student for this instruction is caused by the pressure of these unfolding latent faculties, crying to be born into consciousness. Then there is that wonderful thing, the Will, which is but faintly understood by those ignorant of the Yogi Philosophy--the Power of the Ego--its birthright from the Absolute.

But while these mental and physical things _belong_ to Man, they are _not_ the Man himself. Before the Man is able to master, control, and direct the things belonging to him--his tools and instruments--he must awaken to a realization of Himself. He must be able to distinguish between the "I" and the "Not I." And this is the first task before the Candidate.

That which is the Real Self of Man is the Divine Spark sent forth from the Sacred Flame. It is the Child of the Divine Parent. It is immortal--Eternal--Indestructible--Invincible. It possesses within itself Power, Wisdom, and Reality. But like the infant that contains within itself the sometime Man, the mind of Man is unaware of its latency and potential qualities, and does not know it. As it awakens and unfolds into the knowledge of its real nature, it manifests its qualities, and realizes what the Absolute has given it. When the Real Self begins to awaken, it sets aside from itself those things which are but appendages to it, but which it, in its half-waking state, had regarded as its Self. Setting aside first this, and then that, it finally discards all of the "Not I," leaving the Real Self free and delivered from its bondage to its appendages. Then it returns to the discarded appendages, and makes use of them.

Sanjay Tewani

In considering the question: "What is the Real Self?" let us first stop to examine what man usually means when he says "I." The lower animals do not possess this "I" sense. They are conscious of the outer world; of their own desires and animal cravings and feelings. But their consciousness has not reached the Self-conscious stage. They are not able to think of themselves as separate entities, and to reflect upon their thoughts. They are not possessed of a consciousness of the Divine Spark--the Ego--the Real Self. The Divine Spark is hidden in the lower forms of life--even in the lower forms of human life--by many sheaths that shut out its light. But, nevertheless, it is there, always. It sleeps within the mind of the savage--then, as he unfolds, it begins to throw out its light. In you, the Candidate, it is fighting hard to have its beams pierce through the material coverings When the Real Self begins to arouse itself from its sleep, its dreams vanish from it, and it begins to see the world as it is, and to recognize itself in Reality and not as the distorted thing of its dreams.

The savage and barbarian are scarcely conscious of the "I." They are but a little above the animal in point of consciousness, and their "I" is almost entirely a matter of the consciousness of the wants of the body; the satisfaction of the appetites; the gratification of the passions; the securing of personal comfort; the expression of lust, savage power, etc. In the savage the lower part of the Instinctive Mind is the seat of the "I." (See "Fourteen Lessons" for explanation of the several mental planes of man.) If the savage could analyze his thoughts he would say that the "I" was the physical body, the said body having certain "feelings," "wants" and "desires." The "I" of such a man is a physical "I," the body representing its form and substance. Not only is this true of the savage, but even among so-called "civilized" men of to-day we find many in this stage. They have developed powers of thinking and reasoning, but they do not "live in their minds" as do some of their brothers. They use their thinking powers for the gratification of their bodily desires and cravings, and really live on the plane of the Instinctive Mind. Such a person may speak of "my mind," or "my soul," not from a high position where he looks upon these things from the standpoint of a Master who realizes his Real Self, but from below, from the point-of-view of the man who lives on the plane of the Instinctive Mind and who sees above _himself_ the higher attributes. To such people the body is the "I."

Their "I" is bound up with the senses, and that which comes to them through the senses. Of course, as Man advances in "culture" and "civilization," his senses become educated, and are satisfied only with more refined things, while the less cultivated man is perfectly satisfied with the more material and gross sense gratifications. Much that we call "cultivation" and "culture" is naught but a cultivation of a more refined form of sense gratification, instead of a real advance in consciousness and unfoldment. It is true that the advanced student and Master is possessed of highly developed senses, often far surpassing those of the ordinary man, but in such cases the senses have been cultivated under the mastery of the Will, and are made servants of the Ego instead of things hindering the progress of the soul--they are made servants instead of masters.

As Man advances in the scale, he begins to have a somewhat higher conception of the "I." He begins to use his mind and reason, and he passes on to the Mental Plane--his mind begins to manifest upon the plane of Intellect. He finds that there is something within him that is higher than the body. He finds that his mind seems more _real_ to him than does the physical part of him, and in times of deep thought and study he is able almost to forget the existence of the body.

In this second stage, Man soon becomes perplexed. He finds problems that demand an answer, but as soon as he thinks he has answered them the problems present themselves in a new phase, and he is called upon to "explain his explanation." The mind, even although not controlled and directed by the Will, has a wonderful range, but, nevertheless, Man finds himself traveling around and around in a circle, and realizes that he is confronted continually by the Unknown. This disturbs him, and the higher the stage of "book learning" he attains, the more disturbed does he become. The man of but little knowledge does not see the existence of many problems that force themselves before the attention of the man of more knowledge, and demand an explanation from him. The tortures of the man who has attained the mental growth that enables him to see the new problems and the impossibility of their answer, cannot be imagined by one who has not advanced to that stage.

The man in this stage of consciousness thinks of his "I" as a mental thing, having a lower companion, the body. He feels that he has advanced, but yet his "I" does not give him the answer to the riddles and questions that perplex him. And he becomes most unhappy. Such men often develop into Pessimists, and consider the whole of life as utterly evil and disappointing--a curse rather than a blessing. Pessimism belongs to this plane, for neither the Physical Plane man or the Spiritual Plane man have this curse of Pessimism. The former man has no such disquieting thoughts, for he is almost entirely absorbed in gratifying his animal nature, while the latter man recognizes his mind as an instrument of himself, rather than as _himself_, and knows it to be imperfect in its present stage of growth. He knows that he has in himself the key to all knowledge— locked up in the Ego--and which the trained mind, cultivated, developed and guided by the awakened will, may grasp as it unfolds. Knowing this the advanced man no longer despairs, and, recognizing his real nature, and his possibilities, as he awakens into a consciousness of his powers and capabilities, he laughs at the old despondent, pessimistic ideas, and discards them like a worn-out garment. Man on the Mental Plane of consciousness is like a huge elephant who knows not his own strength. He could break down barriers and assert himself over nearly any condition or environment, but in his ignorance of his real condition and power he may be mastered by a puny driver, or frightened by the rustling of a piece of paper.

When the Candidate becomes an Initiate--when he passes from the purely Mental Plane on to the Spiritual Plane--he realizes that the "I," the Real Self--is something higher than either body or mind, and that both of the latter may be used as tools and instruments by the Ego or "I." This knowledge is not reached by purely intellectual reasoning, although such efforts of the mind are often necessary to help in the unfoldment, and the Masters so use it. The real knowledge, however, comes as a special form of consciousness. The Candidate becomes "aware" of the real "I," and this consciousness being attained, he passes to the rank of the Initiates. When the Initiate passes the second degree of consciousness, and begins to grow into a realization of his relationship to the Whole-- when he begins to manifest the Expansion of Self--then is he on the road to Mastership.

In the present lesson we shall endeavor to point out to the Candidate the methods of developing or increasing the realization of this "I" consciousness--this first degree work. We give the following exercises or development drills for the Candidate to practice. He will find that a careful and conscientious following of these directions will tend to unfold in him a sufficient degree of the "I" consciousness, to enable him to enter into higher stages of development and power. All that is necessary is for the Candidate to feel within himself the dawn of the awakening consciousness, or awareness of the Real Self. The higher stages of the "I" consciousness come gradually, for once on the Path there is no retrogression or going backward. There may be pauses on the journey, but there is no such thing as actually losing that which is once gained on The Path.

This "I" consciousness, even in its highest stages, is but a preliminary step toward what is called "Illumination," and which signifies the awakening of the Initiate to a realization of his actual connection with and relation to the Whole. The full sight of the glory of the "I," is but a faint reflected glow of "Illumination." The Candidate, once that he enters fully into the "I" consciousness, becomes an "Initiate." And the Initiate who enters into the dawn of Illumination takes his first step upon the road to Mastery. The Initiation is the awakening of the soul to knowledge of its real existence--the Illumination is the revelation of the real nature of the soul, and of its relationship with the Whole.

After the first dawn of the "I" consciousness has been attained, the Candidate is more able to grasp the means of developing the consciousness to a still higher degree--is more able to use the powers latent within him; to control his own mental states; to manifest a Centre of Consciousness and Influence that will radiate into the outer world which is always striving and hunting for such centers around which it may revolve.

Man must master himself before he can hope to exert an influence beyond himself. There is no royal road to unfoldment and power--each step must be taken in turn, and each Candidate must take the step himself, and by his own effort. But he may, and will, be aided by the helping hand of the teachers who have traveled The Path before him, and who know just when that helping hand is needed to lift the Candidate over the rough places.

We bid the Candidate to pay strict attention to the following instruction, as it is all important. Do not slight any part of it, for we are giving you only what is necessary, and are stating it as briefly as possible. Pay attention, and follow the instruction closely. This lesson must be mastered before you progress. And it must be practiced not only now, but at many stages of the journey, until full Initiation and Illumination is yours.

Chapter 1- Raja Yoga- The Initiation Process

The first instruction along the line of Initiation is designed to awaken the mind to a full realization and consciousness of the individuality of the "I." The Candidate is taught to relax his body, and to calm his mind and to meditate upon the "I" until it is presented clearly and sharply before the consciousness. We herewith give directions for producing the desired physical and mental condition, in which meditation and concentration are more readily practiced. This state of Meditation will be referred to in subsequent exercises, so the Candidate is advised to acquaint himself thoroughly with it.

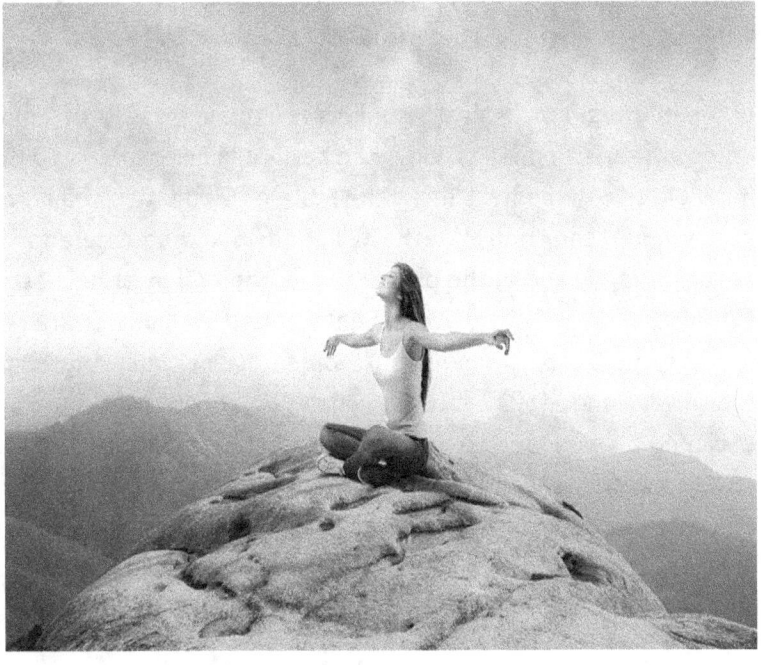

State of Meditation

If possible, retire to a quiet place or room, where you do not fear interruption, so that your mind may feel secure and at rest. Of course, the ideal condition cannot always be obtained, in which case you must do the best you can. The idea is that you should be able to abstract yourself, so far as is possible, from distracting impressions, and you should be alone with yourself--in communion with your Real Self.

It is well to place yourself in an easy chair, or on a couch, so that you may relax the muscles and free the tension of your nerves. You should be able to "let go" all over, allowing every muscle to become limp, until a feeling of perfect peace and restful calm permeates every particle of your being. Rest the body and calm the mind. This condition is best in the early stages of the practice, although after the Candidate has acquired a degree of mastery he will be able to obtain the physical relaxation and mental calm whenever and wherever he desires.

But he must guard against acquiring a "dreamy" way of going around, wrapped in meditation when he should be attending to the affairs of life. _Remember this_, the State of Meditation should be entirely under the control of the Will, and should be entered into only deliberately and at the proper times. The Will must be master of this, as well as of every other mental state. The Initiates are not "day dreamers," both men and women having full control of themselves and their moods. The "I" consciousness while developed by meditation and consciousness, soon becomes a fixed item of consciousness, and does not have to be produced by meditation. In time of trial, doubt, or trouble, the consciousness may be brightened by an effort of the Will (as we shall explain in subsequent lessons) without going into the State of Meditation.

The Realization of the "I"

Sanjay Tewani

The Candidate must first acquaint himself with the reality of the "I," before he will be able to learn its real nature. This is the first step. Let the Candidate place himself in the State of Meditation, as heretofore described. Then let him concentrate his entire attention upon his Individual Self, shutting out all thought of the outside world, and other persons. Let him form in his mind the idea of himself as a _real_ thing--an actual being--an individual entity--a Sun around which the world revolves. He must see himself as the Centre around which the whole world revolves. Let not a false modesty or sense of depreciation interfere with this idea, for you are not denying the right of others to also consider themselves centers. You are, in fact, a center of consciousness--made so by the Absolute--and you are awakening to the fact. Until the Ego recognizes itself as a Centre of Thought, Influence and Power, it will not be able to _manifest_ these qualities. And in proportion as it recognizes its position as a center, so will it be able to manifest its qualities.

It is not necessary that you should compare yourself with others, or imagine yourself greater or higher than them. In fact, such comparisons are to be regretted, and are unworthy of the advanced Ego, being a mark and indication of a lack of development, rather than the reverse. In the Meditation simply ignore all consideration of the respective qualities of others, and endeavor to realize the fact that YOU are a great Centre of Consciousness--a Centre of Power--a Centre of Influence--a Centre of Thought. And that's like the planets circling around the sun, so does your world revolve around YOU who are its center. It will not be necessary for you to argue out this matter, or to convince yourself of its truth by intellectual reasoning. The knowledge does not come in that way. It comes in the shape of a realization of the truth gradually dawning upon your consciousness through meditation and concentration. Carry this thought of yourself as a

"Center of Consciousness--Influence--Power" with you, _for it is an occult truth,_ and in the proportion that you are able, to realize it so will be your ability to manifest the qualities named. No matter how humble may be your position--no matter how hard may be your lot--no matter how deficient in educational advantages you may be—still you would not change your "I" with the most fortunate, wisest and highest man or woman in the world. You may doubt this, but think for a moment and you will see that we are right. When you say that you "would like to be" this person or that, you really mean that _you_ would like to have their degree of intelligence, power, wealth, position, or what not. What you want is something that is theirs, or something akin to it. But you would not for a moment wish to merge your _identity_ with theirs, or to exchange _selves_. Think of this for a moment to _be_ the other person you would have to let _yourself_ die, and instead of _yourself_ you would be the other person. The real _you_ would be wiped out of existence, and you would not be _you_ at all, but would be _he_.

If you can but grasp this idea you will see that not for a moment would you be willing for such an exchange. Of course, such an exchange is impossible. The "I" of you cannot be wiped out. It is eternal, and will go on, and on, and on, to higher and higher states--but it always will be the same "I." Just as you, although a far different sort of person from your childhood self, still you recognize that the same "I" is there and always has been there. And although you will attain knowledge, experience, power and wisdom in the coming years, the same "I" will be there. The "I" is the Divine Spark and cannot be extinguished.

The majority of people in the present stage of the race development have but a faint conception of the reality of the "I." They accept the statement of its existence, and are conscious of themselves as an eating, sleeping, living creature--something like a higher form of animal. But they have not awakened to an "awareness" or realization of the "I," which must come to all who become real centers of Influence and Power. Some men have stumbled into this consciousness, or a degree of it, without understanding the matter. They have "felt" the truth of it, and they have stepped out from the ranks of the commonplace people of the world, and have become powers for good or bad. This is unfortunate to some extent, as this "awareness" without the knowledge that should accompany it may bring pain to the individual and others.

The Candidate must meditate upon the "I," and recognize it--_feel_ it—to be a Centre. This is his first task. Impress upon your mind the word "I," in this sense and understanding, and let it sink deep down into your consciousness, so that it will become a part of you. And when you say "I," you must accompany the word with the picture of your Ego as a Centre of Consciousness, and Thought, and Power, and Influence. See yourself thus, surrounded by your world. Wherever you go, there goes the Centre of your world. YOU are the Centre, and all outside of you revolves around that Centre. This is the first great lesson on the road to Initiation.

Learn It!

The Yogi Masters teach the Candidates that their realization of the "I" as a Centre may be hastened by going into the Silence, or State of Meditation, and repeating their first name over slowly, deliberately and solemnly a number of times. This exercise tends to cause the mind to center upon the "I," and many cases of dawning Initiation have resulted from this practice. Many original thinkers have stumbled upon this method, without having been taught it. A noted example is that of Lord Tennyson, who has written that he attained a degree of Initiation in this way. He would repeat his own name, over and over, and the same time meditating upon his identity, and he reports that he would become conscious and "aware" of his reality and immortality--in short would recognize himself as a _real_ center of consciousness.

We think we have given you the key to the first stage of meditation and concentration. Before passing on, let us quote from one of the old Hindu Masters. He says, regarding this matter: "When the soul sees itself as a Center surrounded by its circumference--when the Sun knows that it is a Sun, and is surrounded by its whirling planets--then is it ready for the Wisdom and Power of the Masters."

CHAPTER 2- INDEPENDENCE OF "I" FROM THE BODY

Many of the Candidates find themselves prevented from a full realization of the "I" (even after they have begun to grasp it) by the confusion of the reality of the "I" with the sense of the physical body. This is a stumbling block that is easily overcome by meditation and concentration, the independence of the "I" often becoming manifest to the Candidate in a flash, upon the proper thought being used as the subject of meditation.

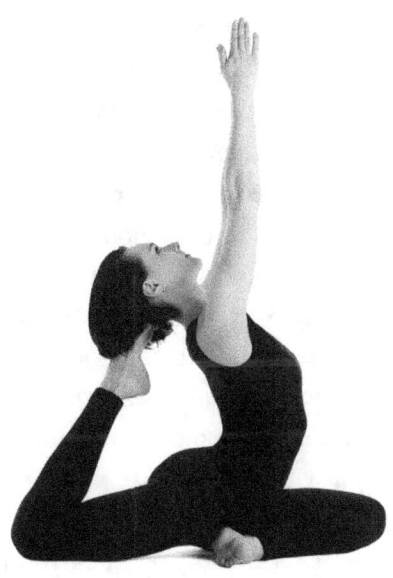

The exercise is given as follows: Place yourself in the State of Meditation, and think of YOURSELF--the Real "I"--as being independent of the body, but using the body as a covering and an instrument. Think of the body as you might of a suit of clothes.

Realize that you are able to leave the body, and still be the same "I." Picture yourself as doing this, and looking down upon your body. Think of the body as a shell from which you may emerge without affecting your identity. Think of yourself as mastering and controlling the body that you occupy, and using it to the best advantage, making it healthy, strong and vigorous, but still being merely a shell or covering for the real "You." Think of the body as composed of atoms and cells which are constantly changing, but which are held together by the force of your Ego, and which you can improve at Will. Realize that you are merely inhabiting the body, and using it for your convenience, just as you might use a house.

In meditating further, ignore the body entirely, and place your thought upon the Real "I" that you are beginning to feel to be "you," and you will find that your identity--your "I"--is something entirely apart from the body. You may now say "my body" with a new meaning. Divorce the idea of your being a physical being, and realize that you are above the body. But do not let this conception and realization cause you to ignore the body.

You must regard the body as the Temple of the Spirit, and care for it, and make it a fit habitation for the "I." Do not be frightened if, during this meditation, you happen to experience the sensation of being out of the body for a few moments, and of returning to it when you are through with the exercise. The Ego is able (in the case of the advanced Initiate) of soaring above the confines of the body, but it never severs its connection at such times. It is merely as if one were to look out of the window of a room, seeing what was going on outside, and drawing in his head when he wishes. He does not leave the room, although he may place his head outside in order to observe what is doing in the street. We do not advise the Candidate to try to cultivate this sensation--but if it comes naturally during meditation, do not fear.

Sanjay Tewani
Realizing the Immortality and Invincibility of the Ego

While the majority accepts on faith the belief in the Immortality of the Soul, yet but few are aware that it may be demonstrated by the soul itself. The Yogi Masters teach the Candidates this lesson, as follows: The Candidate places himself in the State of Meditation, or at least in a thoughtful frame of mind, and then endeavors to "imagine" himself as "dead"—that is, he tries to form a mental conception of himself as dead. This, at first thought, appears a very easy thing to imagine, but as a matter of fact, it is _impossible_ to do so, for the Ego refuses to entertain the proposition, and finds it impossible to imagine it. Try it for yourself.

You will find that you may be able to imagine your _body_ as lying still and lifeless, but the same thought finds that in so doing _You_ are standing and looking at the body. So you see that _You_ are not dead at all, even in imagination, although the body may be. Or, if you refuse to disentangle yourself from your body, in imagination, you may think of your body as dead, but _You_ who refuse to leave it are still _alive_ and recognize the dead body as a thing apart from your Real Self. No matter how you may twist it you _cannot_ imagine yourself as dead.

The Ego insists upon being _alive_ in any of these thoughts, and thus finds that it has within itself the sense and assurance of Immortality. In the case of sleep or stupor resulting from a blow, or from narcotics or anesthetics, the mind is apparently blank, but the "I" is conscious of a continuity of existence. And so one may imagine himself as being in an unconscious state, or asleep, quite easily, and sees the possibility of such a state, but when it comes to imagining the "I" as dead, the mind utterly refuses to do the work. This wonderful fact that the soul carries within itself the evidence of its own immortality is a glorious thing, but one must have reached a degree of unfoldment before he is able to grasp its full significance.

The Candidate is advised to investigate the above statement for himself, by meditation and concentration, for in order that the "I" may know its true nature and possibilities, it must realize that it cannot be destroyed or killed. It must know what it is before it is able to manifest its nature. So do not leave this part of the teaching until you have mastered it. And it is well occasionally to return to it, in order that you may impress upon the mind the fact of your immortal and eternal nature. The mere glimmering of this conception of truth will give you an increased sense of strength and power, and you will find that your Self has expanded and grown, and that you are more of a power and Centre than you have heretofore realized.

The following exercises are useful in bringing about a realization of the invincibility of the Ego--its superiority to the elements. Place yourself in the State of Meditation, and imagine the "I" as withdrawn from the body. See it passing through the tests of air, fire and water unharmed. The body being out of the way, the soul is seen to be able of passing through the air at will--of floating like a bird—of soaring--of traveling in the ether. It may be seen as able to pass through fire without harm and without sensation, for the elements affect only the physical body, not the Real "I." Likewise, it may be seen as passing through water without discomfort or danger or hurt.

This meditation will give you a sense of superiority and strength, and will show you something of the nature of the real "I." It is true that you are confined in the body, and the body may be affected by the elements, but the knowledge that the Real "I" is superior to the body--superior to the elements that affect the body--and cannot be injured any more than it can be killed, is wonderful, and tends to develop the full "I" consciousness within you. For You--the real "I"—are not body. You are Spirit. The Ego is immortal and invincible, and cannot be killed and harmed. When you enter into this realization and consciousness, you will feel an influx of strength and power impossible to describe. Fear will fall from you like a worn-out cloak, and you will feel that you are "born again." An understanding of this thought will show you that the things that we have been fearing cannot affect the Real "I," but must rest content with hurting the physical body. And they may be warded off from the physical body by a proper understanding and application of the Will.

In our next lesson, you will be taught how to separate the "I" from the mechanism of the mind--how you may realize your mastery of the mind, just as you now realize your independence of the body. This knowledge must be imparted to you by degrees, and you must place your feet firmly upon one round of the ladder before you take the next step.

The watchword of this First Lesson is "I." And the Candidate must enter fully into its meaning before he is able to progress. He must realize his real existence--independent of the body. He must see himself as invincible and impervious to harm, hurt, or death. He must see himself as a great Centre of Consciousness--a Sun around which his world revolves. Then will come to him a new strength. He will feel a calm dignity and power, which will be apparent to those with whom he comes in contact. He will be able to look the world in the face without flinching, and without fear, for he will realize the nature and power of the "I." He will realize that he is a Centre of Power--of Influence. He will realize that nothing can harm the "I," and that no matter how the storms of life may dash upon the personality, the real "I"--the Individuality--is unharmed.

Like a rock that stands steadfast throughout the storm, so does the "I" stand through the tempests of the life of the personality. And he will know that as he grows in the realization, he will be able to control these storms and bid them be still.

In the words of one of the Yogi Masters: "The 'I' is eternal. It passes unharmed through the fire, the air, the water. Sword and spear cannot kill or wound it. It cannot die. The trials of the physical life are but as dreams to it. Resting secure in the knowledge of the 'I,' Man may smile at the worst the world has to offer, and raising his hand, he may bid them disappear into the mist from which they emerged. Blessed is he who can say (understandingly) 'I'."

So Dear Candidate, we leave you to master, the First Lesson. Be not discouraged if your progress be slow. Be not cast down if you slip back a step after having gained it. You will gain two at the next step. Success and realization will be yours.

Mastery is before. You will attain. You will accomplish. Peace be with you.

Mantrams (Affirmations) For this Lesson

"I" am a Centre. Around me revolves my world.

"I" am a Centre of Influence and Power.

"I" am a Centre of Thought and Consciousness.

"I" am Independent of the Body.

"I" am Immortal and cannot be destroyed.

"I" am Invincible and cannot be injured.

Chapter 3- The Mental Tools of Ego

In the First Lesson we gave instruction and exercises designed to awaken the consciousness of the Candidate to a realization of the real "I." We confined our instructions to the preliminary teachings of the reality of the "I," and the means whereby the Candidate might be brought to a realization of his real Self, and its independence from the body and the things of the flesh. We tried to show you how you might awaken to a consciousness of the reality of the "I"; its real nature; its independence of the body; its immortality; its invincibility and invulnerability. How well we have succeeded may be determined only by the experience of each Candidate, for we can but point out the way, and the Candidate must do the real work himself.

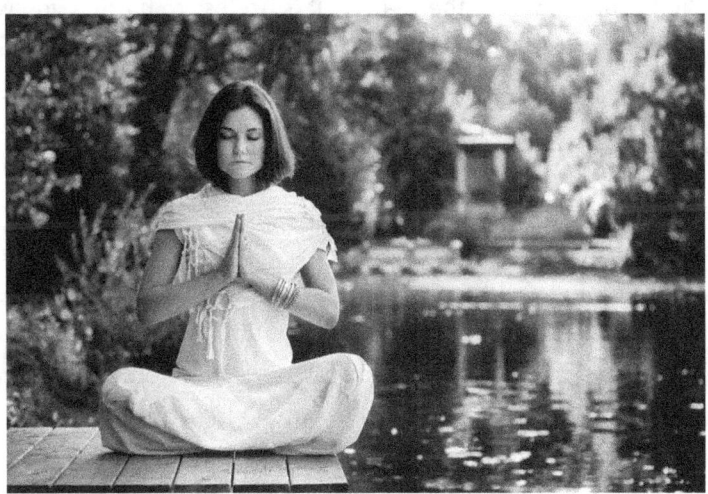

But there is more to be said and done in this matter of awakening to a realization of the "I." So far, we have but told you how to distinguish between the material coverings of the Ego and the "I"

itself. We have tried to show you that you had a real "I," and then to show you what it was, and how it was independent of the material coverings, etc. But there is still another step in this self-analysis--a more difficult step. Even when the Candidate has awakened to a realization of his independence of the body, and material coverings, he often confounds the "I" with the lower principles of the mind. This is a mistake. The Mind, in its various phases and planes, is but a tool and instrument of the "I," and is far from being the "I" itself.

We shall try to bring out this fact in this lesson and its accompanying exercises. We shall avoid, and pass by, the metaphysical features of the case, and shall confine ourselves to the Yogi Psychology. We shall not touch upon theories, nor attempt to explain the cause, nature and purpose of the Mind--the working tool of the Ego--but instead shall attempt to point out a way whereby you may analyze the Mind and then determine which is the "not I" and which is the real "I." It is useless to burden you with theories or metaphysical talk, when the way to prove the thing is right within your own grasp. By using the mind, you will be able to separate it into its parts, and force it to give you its own answer to the questions touching itself.

First, there is what is known as the Instinctive Mind, which man shares in common with the lower animals. It is the first principle of mind that appears in the scale of evolution. In its lower phases, consciousness is but barely perceptible, and mere sensation is apparent. In its higher stages, it almost reaches the plane of Reason or Intellect; in fact, they overlap each other, or, rather, blend into each other. The Instinctive Mind does valuable work in the direction of maintaining animal life in our bodies, it has charge of this part of our being. It attends to the constant work of repair; replacement; change; digestion; assimilation; elimination, etc., all of which work is performed below the plane of consciousness.

But this is but a small part of the work of the Instinctive Mind. For this part of the mind has stored up all the experiences of us and ancestors in our evolution from the lower forms of animal life into the present stage of evolution. All of the old animal instincts (which were all right in their place, and quite necessary for the well-being of the lower forms of life) have left traces in this part of the mind, which traces are apt to come to the front under pressure of unusual circumstances, even long after we think we have outgrown them.

In this part of the mind are to be found traces of the old fighting instinct of the animal; all the animal passions; all the hate, envy, jealousy, and the rest of it, which are our inheritance from the past. The Instinctive Mind is also the "habit mind" in which is stored up all the little, and great, habits of many lives, or rather such as have not been entirely affected by subsequent habits of a stronger nature. The Instinctive Mind is a queer storehouse, containing quite a variety of objects, many of them very good in their way, but others of which are the worst kind of old junk and rubbish.

This part of the mind also is the seat of the appetites; passions; desires; instincts; sensations; feelings and emotions of the lower order, manifested in the lower animals; primitive man; the barbarian; and the man of today, the difference being only in the degree of control over them that has been gained by the higher parts of the mind. There are higher desires, aspirations, etc., belonging to a higher part of the mind, which we will describe in a few minutes, but the "animal nature" belongs to the Instinctive Mind. To it also belong the "feelings" belonging to our emotional and passion nature. All animal desires, such as hunger and thirst; sexual desires (on the physical plane); all passions, such as physical love; hatred; envy; malice; jealousy; revenge, etc., is part of this part of the mind. The desire for the physical (unless a means of reaching higher things) and the longing for the material, belong to this region of the mind. The "lust of the flesh; the lust of the eyes; the pride of life," belongs to the Instinctive Mind.

Take note, however, that we are not condemning the things belonging to this plane of the mind. All of them have their place-- many were necessary in the past, and many are still necessary for the continuance of physical life. All are right in their place, and to those in the particular plane of development to which they belong, and are wrong only when one is mastered by them, or when he returns to pick up an unworthy thing that has been cast off in the unfoldment of the individual.

This lesson has nothing to do with the right and wrong about these things (we have treated of that elsewhere) and we mention this part of the mind that you may understand that you have such a thing in your mental make-up, and that you may understand the thought, etc., coming from it, when we start in to analyze the mind in the latter part of this lesson. All we will ask you to do at this stage of the lesson is to realize that this part of the mind, while _belonging_ to you, is _not_ you, yourself. It is _not_ the "I" part of you.

Next in order, above the Instinctive Mind, is what we have called the Intellect, that part of the mind that does our reasoning, analyzing; "thinking," etc. You are using it in the consideration of this lesson. But note this: You are _using_ it, but it is _not_ You, any more than was the Instinctive Mind that you considered a moment ago. You will begin to make the separation, if you will think but a moment. We will not take up your time with a consideration of Intellect or Reason. You will find a good description of this part of the mind in any good elementary work on Psychology. Our only idea in mentioning it is that you may make the classification, and that we may afterward show you that the

Intellect is but a tool of the Ego, instead of being the real "I" itself, as so many seem to imagine.

The third, and highest, Mental Principle is what is called the Spiritual Mind, that part of the mind which is almost unknown to many of the races, but which has developed into consciousness with nearly all who read this lesson, for the fact that the subject of this lesson attracts you is a proof that this part of your mental nature is unfolding into consciousness. This region of the mind is the source of that which we call "genius," "inspiration," "spirituality," and all that we consider the "highest" in our mental makeup. All the great thoughts and ideas float into the field of consciousness from this part of the mind. All the great unfoldment of the race comes from there. All the higher mental ideas that have come to Man in his upward evolutionary journey, that tend in the direction of nobility; true religious feeling; kindness; humanity; justice; unselfish love; mercy; sympathy, etc., have come to him through his slowly unfolding Spiritual Mind. His love of God and of his fellow man has come in this way. His knowledge of the great occult truths reaches him through this channel. The mental realization of the "I," which we are endeavoring to teach in these lessons, must come to him by way of the Spiritual Mind unfolding its ideas into his field of consciousness.

But even this great and wonderful part of the mind is but a tool—a highly finished one, it is true, but still a tool--to the Ego, or "I."

We propose to give you a little mental drill work, toward the end that you may be able more readily to distinguish the "I" from the mind, or mental states. In this connection we would say that every part, plane, and function of the mind is good, and necessary, and the student must not fall into the error of supposing that because we tell him to set aside first this part of the mind and then that part, that we are undervaluing the mind, or that we regard it as an encumbrance or hindrance. Far from this, we realize that it is _by the use of_ the mind that Man is enabled to arrive at the knowledge of his true nature and self, and that his progress through many stages yet will depend upon the unfolding of his mental faculties.

Man is now using but the lower and inferior parts of his mind, and he has within his mental world great unexplored regions that far surpass anything of which the human mind has dreamed. In fact, it is part of the business of "Raja Yoga" to aid in unfolding these higher faculties and mental regions. And so, far from decrying the Mind, the "Raja Yoga" teachers are chiefly concerned with recognizing the Mind's power and possibilities, and directing the student to avail himself of the latent powers that are inherent in his soul.

It is only by the mind that the teachings we are now giving you may be grasped and understood, and used to your advantage and benefit. We are talking direct to your mind now, and are making appeals to it, that it may be interested and may open itself to what is ready to come into it from its own higher regions. We are appealing to the Intellect to direct its attention to this great matter that it may interpose less resistance to the truths that are waiting to be projected from the Spiritual Mind, which knows the Truth.

Mental Exercise

Place yourself in a calm, restful condition that you may be able to meditate upon the matters that we shall place before you for consideration. Allow the matters presented to meet with a hospitable reception from you, and hold a mental attitude of willingness to receive what may be waiting for you in the higher regions of your mind.

Sanjay Tewani

We wish to call your attention to several mental impressions or conditions, one after another, in order that you may realize that they are merely something _incident_ to you, and _not_ YOU yourself--that you may set them aside and consider them, just as you might anything that you have been using. You cannot set the "I" aside and so consider it, but the various forms of the "not I" may be so set aside and considered.

In the First Lesson you gained the perception of the "I" as independent from the body, the latter merely being an instrument for use. You have now arrived at the stage when the "I" appears to you to be a mental creature--a bundle of thoughts, feelings, moods, etc. But you must go further. You must be able to distinguish the "I" from these mental conditions, which are as much tools as is the body and its parts. Let us begin by considering the thoughts more closely connected with the body, and then work up to the higher mental states.

The sensations of the body, such as hunger; thirst; pain; pleasurable sensations; physical desires, etc., etc., are not apt to be mistaken for essential qualities of the "I" by many of the Candidates, for they have passed beyond this stage, and have learned to set aside these sensations, to a greater or lesser extent, by an effort of the Will, and are no longer slaves to them. Not that they do not experience these sensations, but they have grown to regard them as incidents of the physical life--good in their place-- but useful to the advanced man only when he has mastered them to the extent that he no longer regards them as close to the "I." And yet, to some people, these sensations are so closely identified with their conception of the "I" that when they think of themselves they think merely of a bundle of these sensations. They are not able to set them aside and consider them as things apart, to be used when necessary and proper, but as things not fastened to the "I."

The more advanced a man becomes the farther off seem these sensations. Not that he does not feel hungry, for instance. Not at all, for he recognizes hunger, and satisfies it within reason, knowing that his physical body is making demands for attention, and that these demands should be heeded. But--mark the difference-- instead of feeling that the "_I_" is hungry the man feels that "_my body_" is hungry, just as he might become conscious that his horse or dog was crying for food insistently. Do you see what we mean?

It is that the man no longer identifies himself--the "I"—with the body, consequently the thoughts which are most closely allied to the physical life seem comparatively "separate" from his "I" conception. Such a man thinks "my stomach, this," or "my leg, that," or "my body, thus," instead of "'I,' this," or "'I' that." He is able, almost automatically, to think of the body and its sensations as things _of_ him, and _belonging to_ him, which require attention and care, rather than as real parts of the "I." He is able to form a conception of the "I" as existing without any of these things- -without the body and its sensations--and so he has taken the first step in the realization of the "I."

Before going on, we ask the students to stop a few moments, and mentally run over these sensations of the body. Form a mental image of them, and realize that they are merely incidents to the present stage of growth and experience of the "I," and that they form no real part of it. They may, and will be, left behind in the Ego's higher planes of advancement. You may have attained this mental conception perfectly, long since, but we ask that to give yourself the mental drill at this time, in order to fasten upon your mind this first step.

Realizing that you are able to set aside, mentally, these sensations- -that you are able to hold them out at arm's length and "consider" them as an "outside" thing, you mentally determine that they are "not I" things, and you set them down in the "not I" collection—the first to be placed there. Let us try to make this still plainer, even at the risk of wearying you by repetitions (for you must get this idea firmly fixed in your mind). To be able to say that a thing is "Not I," you must realize that there are two things in question (1) the "not I" thing, and (2) the "I" who is regarding the "Not I" thing just as the "I" regards a lump of sugar, or a mountain. Do you see what we mean? Keep at it until you do.

Next, consider some of the emotions, such as anger; hate; love, in its ordinary forms; jealousy; ambition; and the hundred and one other emotions that sweep through our brains. You will find that you are able to set each one of these emotions or feelings aside and study it; dissect it; analyze it; consider it. You will be able to understand the rise, progress and end of each of these feelings, as they have come to you, and as you recall them in your memory or imagination, just as readily as you would were you observing their occurrence in the mind of a friend. You will find them all stored away in some parts of your mental make-up, and you may (to use a modern American slang phrase) "make them trot before you, and show their paces." Don't you see that they are not "You"—that they are merely something that you carry around with you in a mental bag. You can imagine yourself as living without them, and still being "I," can you not?

And the very fact that you are able to set them aside and examine and consider them is a proof that they are "not I" things--for there are two things in the matter (1) _You_ who are examining and considering them, and (2) the thing itself which is the _object_ of the examination and consideration at mental arm's length. So into the "not I" collection goes these emotions, desirable and undesirable. The collection is steadily growing, and will attain quite formidable proportions after a while.

Now, do not imagine that this is a lesson designed to teach you how to discard these emotions, although if it enables you to get rid of the undesirable ones, so much the better. This is not our object, for we bid you place the desirable (at this time) ones in with the opposite kind, the idea being to bring you to a realization that the "I" is higher, above and independent of these mental things, and then when you have realized the nature of the "I," you may return and use (as a Master) the things that have been using you as a slave. So do not be afraid to throw these emotions (good and bad) into the "not I" collection. You may go back to them, and use the good ones, after the Mental Drill is over. No matter how much you may think that you are bound by any of these emotions, you will realize, by careful analysis, that it is of the "not I" kind, for the "I" existed before the emotion came into active play, and it will live long after the emotion has faded away. The principal proof is that you are able to hold it out at arm's length and examine it--a proof that it is "not I."

Run through the entire list of your feelings; emotions; moods; and what not, just as you would those of a well-known friend or relative, and you will see that each one--every one--is a "not I" thing, and you will lay it aside for the time, for the purpose of the scientific experiment, at least.

Then passing on to the Intellect, you will be able to hold out for examination each mental process and principle. You don't believe it, you may say. Then read and study some good work on Psychology and you will learn to dissect and analyze every intellectual process--and to classify it and place it in the proper pigeonhole. Study Psychology by means of some good textbook, and you will find that one by one every intellectual process is classified, and talked about and labeled, just as you would a collection of flowers.

If that does not satisfy you, turn the leaves of some work on Logic, and you will admit that you may hold these intellectual processes at arm's length and examine them, and talk about them to others. So that these wonderful tools of Man--the Intellectual powers may be placed in the "not I" collection, for the "I" is capable of standing aside and viewing them--it is able to detach them from itself. The most remarkable thing about this is that in admitting this fact, you realize that the "I" is using these very intellectual faculties to pass upon them. Who is the Master that compels these faculties to do this to themselves? The Master of the Mind--The "I."

And reaching the higher regions of the mind--even the Spiritual Mind, you will be compelled to admit that the things that have come into consciousness from that region may be considered and studied, just as may be any other mental thing, and so even these high things must be placed in the "not I" collection. You may object that this does not prove that all the things in the Spiritual Mind may be so treated--that there may be "I" things there that cannot be so treated. We will not discuss this question, for you know nothing about the Spiritual Mind except as it has revealed itself to you, and the higher regions of that mind are like the mind of a God, when compared to what _you_ call mind. But the evidence of the Illumined--those in whom the Spiritual Mind has wonderfully unfolded tell us that even in the highest forms of development, the Initiates, yea, even the Masters, realize that above even their highest mental states there is always that eternal "I" brooding over them, as the Sun over the lake; and that the highest conception of the "I" known even to advanced souls, is but a faint reflection of the "I" filtering through the Spiritual Mind, although that Spiritual Mind is as clear as the clearest crystal when compared with our comparatively opaque mental states. And the highest mental state is but a tool or instrument of the "I," and is not the "I" itself.

And yet the "I" is to be found in the faintest forms of consciousness, and animates even the unconscious life. The "I" is always the same, but its apparent growth is the result of the mental unfoldment of the individual. As we described it in one of the lessons of the "_Advanced Course_" it is like an electric lamp that is encased in many wrappings of cloth. As cloth after cloth is removed, the light seems to grow brighter and stronger, and yet it has changed not, the change being in the removal of the confining and bedimming coverings.

We do not expect to make you realize the "I" in all its fullness--that is far beyond the highest known to man of to-day--but we do hope to bring you to a realization of the highest conception of the "I," possible to each of you in your present stage of unfoldment, and in the process we expect to cause to drop from you some of the confining sheaths that you have about outgrown. The sheaths are ready for dropping, and all that is required is the touch of a friendly hand to cause them to fall fluttering from you. We wish to bring you to the fullest possible (to you) realization of the "I," in order to make an Individual of you--in order that you may understand, and have courage to take up the tools and instruments lying at your hand, and do the work before you.

And now, back to the Mental Drill. After you have satisfied yourself that about everything that you are capable of thinking about is a "not I" thing--a tool and instrument for your use--you will ask, "And now, what is there left that should not be thrown in the "not I" collection." To this question we answer "THE 'I' ITSELF." And when you demand a proof we say, "Try to set aside the 'I' for consideration!"

You may try from now until the passing away of infinities of infinities, and you will never be able to set aside the real "I" for consideration. You may think you can, but a little reflection will show you that you are merely setting aside some of your mental qualities or faculties. And in this process what is the "I" doing? Simply setting aside and considering things. Can you not see that the "I" cannot be both the _considerer_ and the thing considered-- the _examiner_ and the thing examined? Can the sunshine upon itself by its own light? You may consider the "I" of some other person, but it is _your_ "I" that is considering. But you cannot, as an "I," stand aside and see yourself as an "I." Then what evidence have we that there is an "I" to us? This: that you are always conscious of being the considerer and examiner, instead of the considered and examined thing--and then, you have the evidence of your consciousness. And what report does this consciousness give us? Simply this, and nothing more: "I AM." That is all that the "I" is conscious of, regarding its true self: "I AM," but that consciousness is worth all the rest, for the rest is but "not I" tools that the "I" may reach out and use.

And so at the final analysis, you will find that there is something that refuses to be set aside and examined by the "I." And that something is the "I" itself--that "I" eternal, unchangeable--that drop of the Great Spirit Ocean--that spark from the Sacred Flame.

Just as you find it impossible to imagine the "I" as dead, so will you find it impossible to set aside the "I" for consideration--all that comes to you is the testimony: "I AM."

If you were able to set aside the "I" for consideration, who would be the one to consider it? Who could consider except the "I" itself, and if it be _here_, how could it be _there?_ The "I" cannot be the "not I" even in the wildest flights of the imagination--the imagination with all its boasted freedom and power, confesses itself vanquished when asked to do this thing.

Oh, students, may you be brought to a realization of what you are. May you soon awaken to the fact that you are sleeping gods--that you have within you the power of the Universe, awaiting your word to manifest in action. Long ages have you toiled to get this far, and long must you travel before you reach even the first Great Temple, but you are now entering into the conscious stage of Spiritual Evolution. No longer will your eyes be closed as you walk the Path. From now on you will begin to see clearer and clearer each step, in the dawning light of consciousness.

You are in touch with all of life, and the separation of your "I" from the great Universal "I" is but apparent and temporary. We will tell you of these things in our Third Lesson, but before you can grasp that you must develop the "I" consciousness within you. Do not lay aside this matter as one of no importance. Do not dismiss our weak explanation as being "merely words, words, words," as so many are inclined to do. We are pointing out a great truth to you. Why not follow the leadings of the Spirit which even now--this moment while you read--is urging you to walk The Path of Attainment? Consider the teachings of this lesson, and practice the Mental Drill until your mind has grasped its significance, then let it sink deep down into your inner consciousness. Then will you be ready for the next lessons, and those to follow.

Practice this Mental Drill until you are fully assured of the _reality_ of the "I" and the _relativity_ of the "not "I" in the mind. When you once grasp this truth, you will find that you will be able to use the mind with far greater power and effect, for you will recognize that it is your tool and instrument, fitted and intended to do your bidding. You will be able to master your moods, and emotions when necessary, and will rise from the position of a slave to a Master.

Sanjay Tewani

Our words seem cheap and poor, when we consider the greatness of the truth that we are endeavoring to convey by means of them. For who can find words to express the inexpressible? All that we may hope to do is to awaken a keen interest and attention on your part, so that you will practice the Mental Drill, and thus obtain the evidence of your own mentality to the truth. Truth is not truth to you until you have proven it in your own experience, and once so proven you cannot be robbed of it, nor can it be argued away from you.

You must realize that in every mental effort You--the "I"--are behind it. You bid the Mind work, and it obeys your Will. You are the Master, and not the slave of your mind. You are the Driver, not the driven. Shake yourself loose from the tyranny of the mind that has oppressed you for so long. Assert yourself, and be free. We will help you in this direction during the course of these lessons, but you must first assert yourself as a Master of your Mind. Sign the mental Declaration of Independence from your moods, emotions, and uncontrolled thoughts, and assert your Dominion over them. Enter into your Kingdom, thou manifestation of the Spirit!

While this lesson is intended primarily to bring clearly into your consciousness the fact that the "I" is a reality, separate and distinct from its Mental Tools, and while the control of the mental faculties by the Will forms a part of some of the future lessons, still, we think that this is a good place to point out to you the advantages arising from a realization of the true nature of the "I" and the relative aspect of the Mind.

Many of us have supposed that our minds were the masters of ourselves, and we have allowed ourselves to be tormented and worried by thoughts "running away" with us, and presenting themselves at inopportune moments. The Initiate is relieved from this annoyance, for he learns to assert his mastery over the

Page | 41

different parts of the mind, and controls and regulates his mental processes, just as one would a fine piece of machinery. He is able to control his conscious thinking faculties, and direct their work to the best advantage, and he also learns how to pass on orders to the subconscious mental region and bid it work for him while he sleeps, or even when he is using his conscious mind in other matters. These subjects will be considered by us in due time, during the course of lessons.

In this connection it may be interesting to read what Edward Carpenter tells of the power of the individual to control his thought processes. In his book "_From Adam's Peak to Eleplumta," in describing his experience while visiting a Hindu Gnani Yogi, he says:

"And if we are unwilling to believe in this internal mastery over the body, we are perhaps almost equally unaccustomed to the idea of mastery over our own inner thoughts and feelings. That a man should be a prey to any thought that chances to take possession of his mind, is commonly among us assumed as unavoidable. It may be a matter of regret that he should be kept awake all night from anxiety as to the issue of a lawsuit on the morrow, but that he should have the power of determining whether he be kept awake or not seems an extravagant demand. The image of an impending calamity is no doubt odious, but it's very odiousness (we say) makes it haunt the mind all the more pertinaciously and it is useless to try to expel it.

"Yet this is an absurd position--for man, the heir of all the ages: hag-ridden by the flimsy creatures of his own brain. If a pebble in our boot torments us, we expel it. We take off the boot and shake it out. And once the matter is fairly understood, it is just as easy to expel an intruding and obnoxious thought from the mind. About this there ought to be no mistake, no two opinions. The thing is obvious, clear and unmistakable. It should be as easy to expel an obnoxious thought from your mind as it is to shake a stone out of your shoe; and till a man can do that it is just nonsense to talk about his ascendancy over Nature, and all the rest of it. He is a mere slave, and prey to the bat-winged phantoms that flit through the corridors of his own brain.

"Yet the weary and careworn faces that we meet by thousands, even among the affluent classes of civilization, testify only too clearly how seldom this mastery is obtained. How rare indeed to meet a _man_! How common rather to discover a creature hounded on by tyrant thoughts (or cares or desires), cowering, wincing under the lash--or perchance priding himself to run merrily in obedience to a driver that rattles the reins and persuades him that he is free--whom we cannot converse with in careless _tete-a-tete_ because that alien presence is always there, on the watch.

"It is one of the most prominent doctrines of Raja Yoga that the power of expelling thoughts, or if need be, killing them dead on the spot, _must_ be attained. Naturally the art requires practice, but like other arts, when once acquired there is no mystery or difficulty about it. And it is worth practicing. It may indeed fairly be said that life only begins when this art has been acquired. For obvious when instead of being ruled by individual thoughts, the whole flock of them in their immense multitude and variety and capacity is ours to direct and dispatch and employ where we list ('for He maketh the winds his messengers and the flaming fire His minister'), life becomes a thing so vast and grand compared with what it was before, that its former condition may well appear almost antenatal.

"If you can kill a thought dead, for the time being, you can do anything else with it that you please. And therefore it is that this power is so valuable. And it not only frees a man from mental torment (which is nine-tenths at least of the torment of life), but it gives him a concentrated power of handling mental work absolutely unknown to him before. The two things are co-relative to each other. As already said this is one of the principles of Raja Yoga.

"While at work, your thought is to be absolutely concentrated in it, undistracted by anything whatever irrelevant to the matter in hand--pounding away like a great engine, with giant power and perfect economy--no wear and tear of friction, or dislocation of parts owing to the working of different forces at the same time. Then when the work is finished, if there is no more occasion for the use of the machine, it must stop, absolutely--stop entirely--no _worrying_ (as if a parcel of boys was allowed to play their devilments with a locomotive as soon as it was in the shed) --and the man must retire into that region of his consciousness where his true self dwells.

"I say the power of the thought-machine itself is enormously increased by this faculty of letting it alone on the one hand, and of using it singly and with concentration on the other. It becomes a true tool, which a master-workman lays down when done with, but which only a bungler carries about with him all the time to show that he is the possessor of it."

We ask the students to read carefully the above quotations from Mr. Carpenter's book, for they are full of suggestions that may be taken up to advantage by those who are emancipating themselves from their slavery to the unmastered mind, and who are now bringing the mind under control of the Ego, by means of the Will.

Our next lesson will take up the subject of the relationship of the "I" to the Universal "I," and will be called the "Expansion of the Self." It will deal with the subject, not from a theoretical standpoint, but from the position of the teacher who is endeavoring to make his students actually _aware_ in their consciousness of the truth of the proposition. In this course we are not trying to make our students past-masters of _theory_, but are endeavoring to place them in a position whereby they may _know_ for themselves, and actually experience the things of which we teach.

Therefore, we urge upon you not to merely rest content with reading this lesson, but, instead, to study and meditate upon the teachings mentioned under the head of "Mental Drill," until the distinctions stand out clearly in your mind, and until you not only _believe_ them to be true, but actually are _conscious_ of the "I" and its Mental Tools. Have patience and perseverance. The task may be difficult, but the reward is great. To become conscious of the greatness, majesty, strength and power of your real being is worth years of hard study. Do you not think so? Then study and practice, hopefully, diligently and earnestly.

Peace be with you.

Mantrams (Affirmations) For This Lesson

"I" am an entity--my mind is my instrument of expression.

"I" exist independent of my mind, and am not dependent upon it for existence or being.

"I" am Master of my mind, not its slave.

"I" can set aside my sensations, emotions, passions, desires, intellectual faculties, and all the rest of my mental collection of tools, as "not I" things--and still there remains something--and that something is "I," which cannot be set aside by me, for it is my very self; my only self; my real self--"I." That which remains after all that may be set aside _is_ set aside is the "I"--Myself--eternal, constant, unchangeable.

ABOUT THE AUTHOR

Sanjay Tewani came to the realization that he had to make a change in his life when he found that he was filled with a lot of dark thoughts. It was not something that he was comfortable doing and he also found that he was hanging out with the wrong set of people. Thankfully, he was able to get out of this situation before he got in too deep.

How did Sanjay do this? Through yoga! He found a mentor in Suresh Sing who was a master in Raja Yoga. He was a diligent student and was soon teaching himself. Sanjay's main aim is to spread the benefits of yoga to all who he can and he finds that writing is a great medium to do so.